BUH-BYE MEDIOCRITY
HELLO
AWESOMENESS!

BUH-BYE MEDIOCRITY HELLO AWESOMENESS!

A PERFECT COMPANION ON YOUR JOURNEY TO LEAVING COMFY MEDIOCRITY BEHIND AND **EMBRACING YOUR AWESOMENESS.**

BETSY MENDEL

BUH-BYE MEDIOCRITY, HELLO AWESOMENESS!

Copyright © 2024, Betsy Mendel

All rights reserved. Reproduction in part or in whole is strictly forbidden without the express written consent of the publisher, with the exception of a brief quotation for review purposes.

ISBNs:
979-8-9914534-0-0 (paperback)
979-8-9914534-1-7 (eBook)

PRAISE
for *Buh-Bye Mediocrity, Hello Awesomeness!*

"This is a

MUST READ

if you want to be

awesome!"

-17x best-selling author
JON GORDON

To all those out there who are struggling to find
their purpose and passion in life along with financial freedom,
this book is for you.

My heartfelt hope is that
Buh-Bye Mediocrity, Hello Awesomeness! will unlock
your true potential and guide you
on the path to financial abundance and purpose
and above all else, happiness.

Enjoy!

TABLE OF CONTENTS

FOREWORD

HAVE YOU EVER HAD THAT LIFELONG FRIEND WHOM you thought you knew inside out? That was Betsy for me. We've been inseparable since forever. Little did I know, she had this incredible talent for writing and a reservoir of wisdom waiting to be tapped. But wow, did she catch me off guard with this revelation! Let me be clear, Betsy is extraordinary, but this revelation was quite the surprise.

As I sat down to read *Buh-Bye Mediocrity, Hello Awesomeness!* I couldn't help but feel a sense of excitement. In a world inundated with self-help books promising overnight transformations, Betsy's refreshing approach stood out like a ray of sunshine.

In this book, Betsy invites you on a journey—one that transcends the ordinary and leads you toward a life of extraordinary fulfilment. With each turn of the page, you'll discover practical wisdom, heartfelt encouragement, and actionable steps to propel you forward on your path to greatness.

What sets *Buh-Bye Mediocrity, Hello Awesomeness!* apart is its simplicity and sincerity. Betsy's words resonate deeply because they come from a place of genuine understanding and empathy. Through her own experiences and insights, she offers a roadmap for transforming your life one step at a time.

As a best-selling author myself, I know the power of a book

to inspire change. *Buh-Bye Mediocrity, Hello Awesomeness!* is more than just a book—it's a catalyst for personal growth, a beacon of hope, and a guide to living your best life.

So, if you're ready to bid farewell to mediocrity and embrace the awesomeness that awaits you, dive into this book with an open heart and a willingness to take action. Trust me; you won't be disappointed.

Kathryn Gordon,
Best-selling author, *Relationship Grit*
Host of *KATHRYN FOR REAL!* Podcast

PROLOGUE

ARE YOU LIVING IN COMFY MEDIOCRITY? ARE YOU JUST getting by? Are you tired of being broke, of not being able to do the things you really want to do because you can't afford to?

Sick of getting up and going to a job that doesn't bring you joy? You are not alone. According to CNBC, "Gallup, in its recently released State of the Global Workplace 2022 report, found that, along with dissatisfaction, workers are experiencing staggering rates of both disengagement and unhappiness. 60% of people reported being emotionally detached at work and 19% as being miserable. Only 33% reported feeling engaged—and that is even lower than 2020."

If you are ready to take a leap of faith and find what makes you want to jump out of bed and get your day started, then read on. If you are ready to do what comes easily and effortlessly to you and achieve financial freedom, then look no further.

If you, like me, know that you are meant for more, meant for greatness, then you have picked up the right book. There are no coincidences in the universe. If your gut led you to this book, honor that, trust your intuition.

It seems like many people I meet want to reach their full potential but don't think it is possible. They are caught up in the struggle. They are either in jobs that they don't enjoy or are doing the nine to five grind so that they can retire comfortably.

Now don't get me wrong, there is nothing wrong with that. But in my opinion, we're here to live our best life ever, and enjoy our life with passion and purpose while creating financial abundance. And personally, I think this is available to everyone.

Maybe you are going to a job you dread and counting down the days until the weekend. The weekend comes . . . *WOOHOO!* But then the dreaded Sunday night. You know what I'm talking about. Sunday night comes, the weekend is over, and worse than that, you have to wake up Monday morning and do it all over again.

STOP!!!

Let's put an end to this cycle. Seriously, say buh-bye to that life and let's figure out what you love to do and what comes naturally to you. And on top of that, what brings you financial abundance. Sound good?

As you read this book, I want you to do some soul-searching, really dig deep. Complete the short exercises at the end of each chapter to gain clarity on what you desire and the avenues to achieve that. We live in an abundant universe. Anything is possible. If you believe it, you can achieve it.

This book is written in bite-size pieces. Consider it a buffet. You would not eat the entire buffet at one time. Take what resonates with you, savor it, digest it. Come back for seconds and thirds. I believe in *you*!!!! You've so got this!

Bon Appétit!

Now without further ado, let's get to it.

DISCLAIMER: I am going to use the word "universe" throughout this book. Feel free to replace it with whatever resonates with you, whether it's Source Energy, Higher Power, God, Jesus, etc.

CHAPTER 1
What Do You Really Want?

"The great secret of getting what you want from life is to know what you want and believe you can have it."
—Norman Vincent Peale

I WANT TO BE **RICH**!!! I WANT TO STAY IN FIVE-STAR hotels, travel the world in first class, eat at the finest restaurants, drink the best wines, tip big, and spoil the people I love most.

To quote Wallace Wattles from his book *The Science of Getting Rich*:

"There is nothing wrong in wanting to get rich. The desire for riches is really the desire for a richer, fuller, and more abundant life and that is praiseworthy."

What do *you* want?

Discovering what you want in life is a personal journey that involves self-reflection, exploration, and a willingness to try new things.

Deciding is the first step. Stop and really think about what you want. Later, we will figure out the *why* and *how*, but right now let's focus on the *what*.

Here are just a few tips to help you on your path to figuring out what you want:

1. **Evaluate your current situation:** Consider your job, your health, your relationships, and your overall happiness. What is serving you? What is no longer serving you? Take time to think about it and make the necessary changes.

2. **Create a plan:** Make a plan to create your dream life. Finish reading this book and completing the simple exercises at the end of each chapter. If I've

done my job, you should be much clearer on what you want than when you started.

3. **Embrace change:** There's no progress without change. It can be scary stepping out of your comfort zone into the unknown. Learn to embrace change and roll with it.

4. **To thine own self be true:** No one knows more about what you want than you. While it is fine to seek outside opinions, in the end you must be true to yourself. You do *you*!

Remember the process of defining what you want is ongoing and it's okay to change course as you go along. Regularly revisit and reassess your aspirations and goals and make sure they still align with you.

Really dig deep and think about what you want in this life. Do you want to:

- Own a house?

- Get married?

- Start a family?

- Make a million dollars?

- Become famous?

Focus on what you want. The sky's the limit.

EXERCISE

I want:

1. To be a best-selling author.

2. To be financially free.

3. To inspire the masses to leave mediocrity behind and awaken their awesomeness.

Now your turn. What do you want:

1.

2.

3.

I am ready.
I am available.
Show me how.

Notes

CHAPTER 2
What Is Your Why?

"When your why is big enough you will find your how."
—Les Brown

WHAT IS YOUR *WHY* AND WHY IS IT SO IMPORTANT TO know? I'm glad you asked. The importance of your *why* is to understand your motivation behind your actions, goals, and decisions.

Your *why* is the core reason that drives you to do what you do. It gives meaning and direction to your life. Your *why* is the driving force behind all that you do. It allows you to prioritize and to let go of what isn't serving you. Some of us know our why, some of us don't, and for some of us, it changes over the course of a lifetime.

Think about what motivates you to get out of bed and start your day? If you know your *why*, that's great! If you are unclear on your *why*, don't fret. Here are some steps you can take to discover your *why*:

1. **Notice what makes you happy:** What brings you joy? What lights your fire? Identifying what you are passionate about can provide valuable clues about your *why*.

2. **Discover your strengths:** Make a list of your strengths and talents. What are you naturally good at? What comes easily to you? Your *why* is often connected to utilizing your strengths and making a meaningful impact through them.

3. **Trust your instincts:** Listen to your gut. Pay atten-

tion to your intuition or that gut feeling you experience in certain situations. Trusting and following these feelings can lead you closer to your *why*.

4. **Don't overthink it:** I'm guilty of this. Overthinking is just another way of procrastinating. Stop overthinking and get to it.

5. **Act now:** Action is the key to success. Just put one foot in front of the other and GET STARTED.

Remember, discovering your *why* is an ongoing process. It may take time, self-reflection, and trial and error to fully understand what motivates you. Embrace the journey, be open to new experiences, and allow your *why* to evolve as you grow and gain new insights.

EXERCISE

My *why*:

1. To live with passion and purpose. To inspire my readers to break free from mediocrity and embrace their awesomeness.

2. To live comfortably, to take care of my family and loved ones, and to travel the world.

3. To look and feel my best every day while encouraging others to do the same.

What's your *why*:

1.

2.

3.

I am ready.
I am available.
Show me how.

Notes

CHAPTER 3
How Now Brown Cow

"You don't have to be great to start,
but you have to start to be great."
—Zig Ziglar

OK GREAT. NOW YOU HAVE IDENTIFIED YOUR WHY. Now the question becomes *how*? This is a tough one and keeps many of us sidelined.

The *how* gets in the way of getting started. We want a step-by-step plan. Having a well-laid-out plan is great, but unfortunately, believing that this is essential holds many of us from taking action.

Think about your GPS. When you plug in your destination, it gives you the next turn. Not all your turns at once but just the very next one. And then once you've completed that one, you get the next one . . . the next step. Same is true for us.

Get a crystal-clear picture in your mind of what you want, and do not dwell on the *how*. Try to really see it, feel it, and be as specific as you can. After all, if you want to go to San Francisco, you don't plug California in your GPS. If you are vague, your GPS will give you vague directions. The same is true with the universe. The more specific and descriptive you are, the better the universe can help you manifest it. Use the following steps to start you on the path to your *how*:

1. **Break it down:** Break things down into smaller, manageable tasks. As the saying goes: "How do you eat an elephant? One bite at a time."

2. **Prioritize and plan:** Which tasks are most important? Make a list and prioritize them. Have a timeline to keep you on track.

3. **Take the first step:** Getting started can be the hardest part. Pick one task from your plan. Complete it. Taking action creates momentum and builds confidence.

4. **Seek guidance and support:** Ask others for advice. Go to Facebook and Instagram and reach out to others that are doing or have done what you want to do. Follow them on social media. Even Direct Message them. You never know.

5. **Stay motivated and persevere:** Taking the first step can be challenging, and setbacks will occur. Stay motivated by reminding yourself of your goal. Post it on your bulletin board or on the dashboard of your car to serve as a reminder when you get caught up and feel like giving up. I'm telling you; I almost shelved this book several times. The advice I got from a good friend really pushed me forward: "You have to take it to the finish line regardless of the outcome."

Get started and trust that the next step will reveal itself in the form of new ideas, surprise opportunities, and people you need to connect with along the way.

EXERCISE

I am going to:

1. Study and hone my craft by reading a chapter of a book that inspires and motivates me daily, brainstorming with friends, following successful authors on social media.

2. Reduce unnecessary spending, cook meals at home, seek out Happy Hours (great way to save money while still going out), pay bills on time (avoid late fees and interest).

3. Move my body daily, follow a plant-based diet, stay positive, get eight hours of sleep a night, meditate on the daily and drink 64oz. of water every day, and lastly, listen to my body.

Think about three things you can do right now:

1.

2.

3.

I am ready.
I am available.
Show me how.

Notes

CHAPTER 4
Uncover Your Unique Gift

"You can do something extraordinary,
and something a lot of people can't do.
And if you have the opportunity to work on your gifts,
it seems like a crime not to. I mean, it's just weakness to quit
because something becomes too hard."
—Morgan Matson

WE ALL HAVE A SPECIAL GIFT THAT WE WERE PUT ON this earth to share. What is your gift? That is the age-old question: Why am I here? What is my purpose? The truth is we all have a path and purpose for being here. Yet, many of us struggle to recognize the special qualities and talents we possess. Sometimes it may feel as though your gift isn't important. But at the end of the day, who you are, what you do and how you show up in the world matters. To illustrate this, I want to share the story of *Kyle* written by Barbara Mikkelson:

"One day, when I was a freshman in high school, I saw a kid from my class was walking home from school. His name was Kyle. It looked like he was carrying all of his books. I thought to myself, 'Why would anyone bring home all his books on a Friday? He must really be a nerd.'

I had quite a weekend planned (parties and a football game with my friends tomorrow afternoon), so I shrugged my shoulders and went on. As I was walking, I saw a bunch of kids running toward him. They ran at him, knocking all his books out of his arms and tripping him so he landed in the dirt. His glasses went flying, and I saw them land in the grass about ten feet from him. He looked up and I saw this terrible sadness in his eyes. My heart went out to him. So, I jogged over to him and as he crawled around looking for his glasses, I saw a tear in his eye.

As I handed him his glasses, I said, 'Those guys are jerks. They really should get lives.' He looked at me and said, 'Hey thanks!' There was a big smile on his face. It was one of those smiles that showed real gratitude.

I helped him pick up his books and asked him where he lived. As it turned out, he lived near me, so I asked him why I had never seen him before. He said he had gone to private school. I would have never hung out with a private school kid before.

We talked all the way home, and I carried his books. He turned out to be a pretty cool kid. I asked him if he wanted to play football on Saturday with me and my friends. He said yes. We hung all weekend and the more I got to know Kyle, the more I liked him. And my friends thought the same of him.

Monday morning came, and there was Kyle with the huge stack of books again. I stopped him and said, 'Damn boy, you are gonna really build some serious muscles with this pile of books every day!' He just laughed and handed me half the books. Over the next four years, Kyle and I became best friends. When we were seniors, we began to think about college. Kyle decided on Georgetown, and I was going to Duke. I knew that we would always be friends, that the miles would never be a problem. He was going to be a doctor, and I was going for business on a football scholarship. Kyle was valedictorian of our class.

I teased him all the time about being a nerd. He had to pre-pare a speech for graduation. I was so glad it wasn't me having to get up there and speak. Graduation day, I saw Kyle.

He looked great. He was one of those guys that really found himself during high school. He filled out and actually looked good in glasses. He had more dates than me and all the girls loved him! Boy, sometimes I was jealous.

Today was one of those days. I could see that he was nervous about his speech. So, I smacked him on the back and said, 'Hey big guy, you'll be great!' He looked at me with one of those looks (the really grateful one) and smiled. 'Thanks,' he said.

As he started his speech, he cleared his throat, and began. 'Graduation is a time to thank those who helped you make it through those tough years. Your parents, your teachers, your siblings, maybe a coach . . . but mostly your friends. I am here to tell all of you that being a friend to someone is the best gift you can give them. I am going to tell you a story.' I just looked at my friend with disbelief as he told the story of the first day we met. He had planned to kill himself over the weekend. He talked of how he had cleaned out his locker so his mom wouldn't have to do it later and was carrying his stuff home. He looked hard at me and gave me a little smile. 'Thankfully, I was saved. My friend saved me from doing the unspeakable.' I heard the gasp go through the crowd as this handsome, popular boy told us all about his weakest moment.

I saw his mom and dad looking at me and smiling that same grateful smile. Not until that moment did I realize its depth. Never underestimate the power of your actions. With one small gesture you can change a person's life."

Sometimes we don't see in ourselves what others can see in us. I know you've been told before "If only you knew how great you are." Am I right? Well, take that a step further. Ask them to let you know what they mean by that. Ask a friend or relative if they could tell you about a gift or talent they see in you. One time I made a brag book for my friend for her birthday. I called several of her friends and asked them what made her special to them. It was amazing what people had to say. I gave the book to my friend, and she cherishes it to this day. If she is having a hard time or feeling bad about herself, she simply pulls out the brag book and reads it.

To uncover your gifts, think about what comes easily and effortlessly to you. For me, I have a special gift of attracting and connecting with people. I make lifetime friends wherever I go. I love people and I love to hear their stories. I love to meet new people, and the universe has blessed me with the gift of attracting and bonding with people.

I know if I put one foot in front of the other, if I suit up and show up, the universe will open all kinds of doors and opportunities for me that I never knew existed.

What's your gift? Remember, *you* matter!

EXERCISE

List three things that come easily and effortlessly to you. Don't worry about how you'll monetize it. Right now, we are just focusing on your special gifts. I'll start:

1. I have a magnetic personality.

2. I have a knack for writing.

3. I'm a natural salesperson.

It can be as simple as that. Now it's your turn:

1.

2.

3.

I am ready.
I am available.
Show me how.

Notes

CHAPTER 5
Dream Big, Really Big

"If you can dream it, you can do it."
—Sheralyn Silverstein

DREAM **BIG**! I MEAN, THINK ABOUT IT . . . THOMAS EDI-son invented the light bulb; Ben Franklin invented the light-ning rod; the Wright Brothers invented the airplane; we put a man on the moon; Elon Musk makes electric cars.

Don't you think those inventions and accomplishments were dreams in their minds before they became a reality? Of course they were! They took the next step and persisted until they achieved their dream.

We've all heard follow your dream and dream big. What does this really mean? Dreaming big is about pushing yourself to be the best *you* that you can be. After all, my dream for writing this book is not to get limited placements around the country. My dream is to become an international best-selling author and to have my books front and center at every book-store and airport kiosk. To become fabulously wealthy to boot. And, of course, to inspire you, my readers, to do the same. Go for it! Give it your all and then some. To quote Neil Armstrong, "Shoot for the stars, but if you happen to miss, shoot for the moon instead."

We live in a universe where anything and everything is pos-sible. I mean, really, Gary Dahl invented the Pet Rock. The fad exploded with more than one million of them selling. And that was in 1975 before the World Wide Web, social media, and Amazon. Imagine what could have happened if all these ave-nues were available back then. I think each of us would have a pet rock sitting on our desk. Anything is possible!!!

What are you waiting for? I know you have dreams simmering inside you. We all do. Go for it! And while you're at it, don't put any limitations on your dreams. Go big or go home!

The future belongs to those who dream big. Here are a few ways to embrace dreaming big:

1. **Think about your ideal future:** Where are you living? What are you doing? Are you living your best life ever? Really visualize the details.

2. **Set ambitious goals:** Set goals that challenge you. Don't be afraid to aim for something that seems impossible. After all, the word impossible says "I'm possible!"

3. **Believe in yourself:** Let me repeat: Believe in yourself. If you don't believe in yourself, who will? Trust in your potential. Surround yourself with positive people who believe in you.

4. **Take consistent action:** Dreams without action is just a wish. Taking consistent, purposeful steps toward your goals every day is key. Even small steps accumulate over time and bring you closer to your dream life.

Remember, dreaming big is not limited to specific areas of your life. You can dream big in your career, personal relationships, fitness, health, as well as making a difference in the world. Embrace the power of your imagination, believe in yourself, and take inspired action to transform your dreams into reality.

So, dig deep, dream big, and see how high you can go! And get ready to live the life of your wildest dreams!

EXERCISE

List three ginormous dreams you have right now. Stretch yourself! No limits! I'll start:

1. This book makes me a best-selling author inspiring people all over the world to become amazingly awesome.

2. I am bicoastal, splitting my time between Atlanta and Santa Monica.

3. People recognize me when I am out and thank me for changing their lives in a positive way.

Now your turn:

1.

2.

3.

I am ready.
I am available.
Show me how.

Notes

CHAPTER 6
Just Ask

"Ask and it is given"
—Esther & Jerry Hicks

I KNOW THERE ARE THINGS YOU DESIRE. WE ALL DO. Just put it out there. *Ask.* If you don't ask, you don't get. A closed mouth doesn't get fed.

I want to become a best-selling author! I want to write books that inspire the masses to live up to their full potential and live their best life ever! I want to become a multimillionaire! See, that wasn't so hard. I asked, I put it out there, and now I'm ready to receive.

Next, you must be specific. Be very, very specific. One of the secrets to getting what you want is knowing what you want. The universe cannot decipher mixed messages. The more specific you are, the more universal something can become. Life is in the details.

I recently decided I wanted to go to Atlanta for a couple of months to visit my 91-year-old mom and to write this book. I asked a friend if she knew of a place I could stay. She said she had a condo in Buckhead that is not being used. And to top it off, Elton John lives in the penthouse of the building. So, not only did I manifest a place to stay, but I manifested an amazing place to stay. I asked and I received. You'd be surprised by how much people really want to help.

The act of asking can be a powerful tool. Here are a couple of reasons why asking can be impactful:

1. **Problem-solving:** When you get stuck, reach out. Get feedback or alternative viewpoints. I had sever-

al friends read the draft of my book to offer suggestions, and I believe it made this a better book.

2. **Building relationships:** People like to help. Don't be shy to ask. Network, make connections. You never know who knows who.

3. **Different point of view:** Everyone sees the world in a different way. By asking you can get another perspective.

Remember, asking thoughtful questions can lead to valuable insights, opportunities, and personal growth. It is an essential skill to develop in both professional and personal realms.

EXERCISE

What will I ask for today:

1. Inspiration, guidance, and insight.

2. Excellent health for me, my loved ones, and the world.

3. To impact as many people as possible to say buh-bye to mediocrity.

Now it's your turn. Remember, it's all in the details.

1.

2.

3.

I am ready.
I am available.
Show me how.

Notes

CHAPTER 7
Obstacles

"Obstacles are those frightful things you see when you take your eyes off your goal."
—Henry Ford

THERE ARE GOING TO BE OBSTACLES IN LIFE. IT'S JUST the nature of the game. Expect them. Overcome them.

I would be remiss if I said I haven't had my share of obstacles. This is the part of the book where I had to decide how vulnerable and raw I really wanted to be. I debated over and over and in the end, I decided to go for it in the hopes of helping others.

Here goes:

For me, life's not been a straight line. I have been thrown my share of curveballs. I have suffered from depression my entire adult life. I was diagnosed with major depressive disorder and I'm here to tell you, it's no walk in the park. Top that off with an eating disorder and an exercise addiction and voilà, you've got a perfect trifecta.

I know what it's like to be in the depths of despair and utter hopelessness. I've been in the trenches and have come out the other side victorious. So, while there are no letters before or after my name, I consider myself an authority as I have lived it. I have fought hard and won the battle. I'm determined to guide you to do the same. I can honestly say I'm proud of the woman I am today because I went through one hell of a time becoming her.

As you can see, depression has been my biggest obstacle in life. I could write another book about that but I'm going to shorten it and say that if you suffer from any of the aforementioned or any other mental health issues, please, please, please seek help. There is no longer a stigma around these conditions. With the help of a psychiatrist and an amazing therapist, I am able to keep things at bay and live a meaningful and productive life.

We all have obstacles and problems in life. When facing problems, do not get discouraged. Remember it's temporary. There is a solution to every problem. I know when you're in the midst of a challenge, it's hard to remember. Use the following tips to help you on your way:

1) **Positive attitude:** Cultivate a positive and optimistic mindset. View obstacles as challenges and opportunities for growth rather than insurmountable barriers.

2) **Results not reasons:** I once had a manager that said this every time you came to him with a problem. Sounds harsh but all it really means is to focus on the solution, not the problem. Try it. It works.

3) **Fail forward:** Failure is often a stepping stone to success. Learn from your mistakes and use failure as an opportunity to improve. Simply put, fail forward.

4) **Focus on what you can control:** Let's face it, there are going to be aspects of a situation that may be beyond your control. Focus your energy on what you can control and let go of what you cannot.

5) **Celebrate progress:** This is one many of us forget about. Acknowledge and celebrate your victories. Recognizing your accomplishments is a great motivation booster. Do something that brings you joy.

I like to go get my favorite boba drink. That makes me happy.

Overcoming obstacles is not always easy but don't give up. Remember to every problem, there is a solution. Find it.

EXERCISE

Since you may not be facing any obstacles right now, save this exercise and fill it in as you encounter an obstacle.

What are three obstacles you are facing right now? What is the solution?

1) Obstacle:

Solution:

2) Obstacle:

Solution:

3) Obstacle:

Solution:

Extra credit: Take your biggest obstacle of the three you just listed and get busy on the solution!

I am ready.
I am available.
Show me how.

Notes

Notes

CHAPTER 8
Be Persistent

*"Never, never, never, never—in nothing, great or small,
large or petty—never give in, except to convictions of
honour and good sense. Never yield to force."*
—Winston Churchill

THIS FAMOUS QUOTE THAT WINSTON CHURCHILL DE-
livered in his commencement speech in 1941 at Harrow School
still holds true today. You must be persistent despite difficulties
or obstacles.

Persistence is the ability to stand up and take a step forward
when everyone else sits down. It is a key ingredient to success.
Without persistence, it doesn't matter how talented you are because your full potential will never be achieved.

People who are persistent are often willing to put in the
necessary effort, time, and energy to achieve their desired out-
comes. They maintain a positive mindset and are resilient in
the face of difficulties. They understand that setbacks and failures are a part of the process and view them as learning opportunities rather than reasons to give up.

Persistence is a valuable trait in various areas of life, including personal goals, professional pursuits, and academic endeav-
ors. It can help individuals overcome obstacles, develop new
skills, and reach higher levels of success. It requires discipline,
patience, and the ability to adapt and adjust strategies when
necessary.

It's not easy to continue when the going gets tough. But
keep going! It will be worth it!

Remember, if everything came easily, we wouldn't know
what it felt like to truly succeed. Obstacles are opportunities
for growth and expansion. It is the nature of the game. But if
you persist and keep your eye on the prize, you can get past any

and all obstacles. I mean, take a look at Abraham Lincoln. He suffered a multitude of failures and setbacks in his life:

Lost his job in 1832
Defeated for state legislature in 1832
Failed in business in 1833
Elected to state legislature in 1834
Sweetheart died in 1835
Had a nervous breakdown in 1836
Defeated for Speaker in 1838
Defeated for nomination for Congress in 1843
Elected to Congress in 1846
Lost renomination in 1848
Rejected for land officer in 1849
Defeated for U.S. Senate in 1854
Defeated for nomination for Vice President in 1856
Again, defeated for U.S. Senate in 1858
Elected President in 1860

Thankfully he persisted and did not let all these setbacks get in his way. Finally, he won the presidency and changed the course of history.

Persistence trumps setbacks every time. Remember, when the going gets tough, the tough get going.

Here are just a couple of ways to get the ball rolling:

1. **Get a role model:** If you reach a gridlock or have a setback (and trust me, you will), get a role model to help you through it. Someone that has been through it before and reached their goal. You would be surprised at how people truly want to help. Reach out! Who better to advise you than someone who has persisted and made it to the finish line.

2. **Join or start a mastermind group:** Gather like-minded people who are determined to be their best. The movers and shakers of the world. Meet once a month or twice a month or whatever works best for the group. It doesn't have to be in person. Virtual groups are a great way to go. There is power in people. You can also Google "mastermind groups near me." Meetup and Facebook are great resources as well.

3. **Have an accountability partner:** An accountability partner can significantly increase your chances of success in achieving your goals by providing structure, support, and motivation throughout your journey.

What are you determined to do with this one short life you have been given? Do you want to change the world? Do you want to become famous? Do you want to be filthy rich?

Determination, hard work, and persistence can move mountains.

Persist, persist, persist!

EXERCISE

I will persist today by:

1. Keeping the end goal in mind.

2. Checking in with my accountability partner when I hit a speed bump.

3. Staying focused on the task at hand.

How will you persist today?

1.

2.

3.

I am ready.
I am available.
Show me how.

Notes

Notes

CHAPTER 9
Routine, Routine, Routine

"Wake up and smell the routine."
—Lance Lang

I CANNOT STRESS ENOUGH THE IMPORTANCE OF HAV-ing and sticking to a routine. A routine is the normal order in which we regularly do things, a habit or sequence that doesn't vary. Just as we get a baby into a routine for feeding and sleeping, we need to do the same for ourselves. Routines create structure and promote mental, physical, and emotional health.

We feel more confident and secure when our daily activities are predictable and familiar. If we do certain things in the same way, it frees our minds to focus on the more important things. Our daily routines can make a huge difference to how healthy, happy, and productive we are. Sticking to a routine requires commitment and dedication. But I promise you, having the structure in place will be a game changer.

Here are some key reasons why routines are so important:

1. **Structure and organization:** Routines provide structure and organization. They help us establish a framework, thereby allowing you to get through your day more efficiently. Knowing what you're going to do, and when, gives you a sense of control over your day, which can significantly reduce stress and anxiety. Routines provide a sense of stability and predictability, allowing us to better manage uncertainties and adapt to changes.

2. **Time management:** Routines can help you manage your time more efficiently. Time blocking, or divid-

ing your day into blocks of time, where each block is dedicated to a specific task is a great tool for managing your day. Instead of keeping an open-ended to-do list of things you will get to when you can, you will have a concrete schedule outlining what you will work on and when. Personally, I like to write mine on a daily calendar.

3. **Healthy habits:** By incorporating activities such as exercise, proper nutrition, self-care, and adequate rest into your routine, you make these behaviors a regular part of your life. This leads to improved physical and mental well-being.

4. **Work-life balance:** Routines can help establish a healthy work-life balance. By setting boundaries and allocating time for work, family, play, and relaxation, we can ensure that all aspects of our lives receive attention and maintain harmony.

Routines contribute to our overall well-being by providing stability, order, and a sense of purpose. They help us lead more balanced, fulfilling lives, and contribute to our long-term happiness and success.

It's worth noting that while routines can be highly beneficial, it's also important to maintain flexibility and adaptability to accommodate unexpected events and changes in circumstances. Recently, I had plans to take a magnificent hike which I had been looking forward to for days. But the weather had another plan. I woke up Saturday morning to a rainstorm. Hey, what's going on here? It's not supposed to rain in Southern California. So, off to the gym I went. Not really what I wanted to do, but I changed my course. I not only had a great workout, but I ran into an old friend who is also writing a book. Coincidence? I think not. Striking a balance between routine and flexibility is key to enjoying the benefits without feeling trapped or limited by rigid schedules.

Here's a step-by-step guide on how to set a routine:

1. **Assess your current schedule:** Look at your current schedule and identify time slots available for building your routine.

2. **Determine time blocks:** Prioritize your activities. Divide your day into time blocks, allocating specific time periods for what must get done. Include work, exercise, hobbies, and family time. Be sure to consider energy levels throughout the day. Listen to your circadian clock. We all have different ones. I get my best work done early in the morning.

3. **Start with small steps:** If you're new to routines, it's helpful to start small. Begin by incorporating a few key activities into your routine, and gradually build on them over time. Trying to make drastic changes all at once can be overwhelming and difficult to sustain.

4. **Stay consistent and track progress:** Consistency is key when it comes to routines. Try to stick to your schedule as much as possible, even on days when you don't feel like it. Track your progress to stay motivated and make any necessary adjustments along the way.

If you don't have a routine in place, now is the perfect time to start. Keep a routine for your sleep, your diet, your exercise, and your work. These are crucial areas to focus on for living a healthy and balanced lifestyle. Remember, this is your life, and you must do it the way that works best for you. Here is what works for me:

5:00am – Jump out of bed (Don't hate me . . . I'm a morning person).

Floss and brush my teeth, mouthwash.

15 second ice cold shower (I'm working my way up to a minute). This shocks the nervous system, and you will be wide awake, trust me.

Next, I jump on my mini trampoline for 20 minutes while listening to my favorite music. (Country, if you must know.) Jumping on the trampoline flushes out my lymphatic system, thereby strengthening my immune system. I would highly recommend investing in one. They are inexpensive and you can find one at your local sporting goods store, or online, of course.

5:45am – Off to the gym to take my favorite 6:00am class.

7:00am – Home to shower.

7:15am – Drink my protein shake. I love a brand called OWYN (Only What You Need). I love the chocolate, and I add mint extract in for extra flavor and MCT oil for brain health.

7:45am – Dress for success (usually means Lululemon tights with a top . . . I have the added bonus of working remotely so that is pretty much my uniform).

8:00am – Write and coach. I'm a Health and Wellness Coach and Personal Trainer along with working toward my goal of becoming a best-selling author.

10:15am – Eat a healthy snack. Always something plant based. Back to work.

12:30pm – Lunchtime. Usually, a hearty salad or a veggie wrap with hummus. Love that!

1:00pm – Back to work.

3:00pm(ish) – 15-minute meditation. I find a comfortable space, put in my AirPods, and go to YouTube for meditation music. This is what works for me. A daily habit of meditation can seem very challenging for some, but the benefits far outweigh the disadvantages. And you can meditate for as little or as long as you like. Heck, even five minutes is a good start.

3:20pm(ish) – Free flow writing and gratitude list.

4:45pm – Back to work.

6:00pm – Eat dinner in the neighborhood. I'm fortunate enough that I can walk down the street and have an awesome array of healthy restaurants. Other nights I cook, experimenting with different plant-based recipes.

7:00pm – I hate to admit what I do next. Don't judge me. I watch mindless (aka Reality) TV. It makes me laugh which in turn releases endorphins, a feel-good hormone.

8:45pm – My eyes start to close and I'm out by 9:00pm. I get a good night's sleep and wake up refreshed, ready to start all over again. Remember what Benjamin Franklin said: "Early to bed, early to rise, makes a man healthy, wealthy, and wise."

Take a moment to think about your daily routine. Is it serving you? Are you all over the board with no structure?

EXERCISE

What does your routine look like right now? To recap, here is mine:

1. Gym first thing in the morning.

2. Fuel my body with healthy food.

3. Going to bed early and waking up early.

What are you consistently doing on a daily basis? Take a minute to really think about it and then list three of them below:

1.

2.

3.

I am ready.
I am available.
Show me how.

Notes

CHAPTER 10
Bright, Shiny Objects

"Be about actions, not distraction."
—Muhammad Tahir Ayoob

THE PHRASE "BRIGHT, SHINY OBJECTS" IS COMMONLY used metaphorically to describe things that capture our attention or distract us, often at the expense of more important or meaningful matters. In this context, it suggests that we may become easily enthralled by superficial or trivial things, diverting our focus from more significant issues.

Metaphorically, the term can also be associated with the concept of shiny object syndrome, where individuals have a tendency to chase after new ideas, trends, or opportunities without thoroughly evaluating their worth or considering the potential consequences. Also known as immediate gratification.

In the world we live in today, there is no shortage of distractions . . . social media, our phones, bright, shiny objects, to name just a few. I am guilty as charged. I consider myself the queen of distractions. As a matter of fact, if you look up the word "distraction" you will see my picture. All joking aside, this is probably my biggest downfall. I can always find something to do besides what needs to be done. Oh, TJ Maxx is around the corner, and I really need ____________. I'm craving my favorite ____________ at the café down the street. __________ called yesterday and I forgot to call her back. You get the gist. What's a woman to do? But men, you don't get off the hook either. You know, the football game starts in an hour, I'm hungry, my car needs to be cleaned. The list can go on and on but here are some of the more common ones:

1. **Mobile devices and social media:** The constant notifications, messages, and access to social media platforms on our smartphones are major distractions. It's easy to get caught up in scrolling through news feeds or engaging in online conversations instead of focusing on work or other important tasks.

2. **Multitasking:** "You can't ride two horses with one ass," gets the point across. Trying to juggle multiple tasks simultaneously can reduce productivity and increase errors because our attention is divided among different activities.

3. **Cluttered environment:** A cluttered or disorganized physical space can be visually distracting and make it harder to concentrate. It's easier to stay focused when your surroundings are tidy and free from unnecessary items.

4. **Interruptions:** Unexpected interruptions, such as phone calls, text messages, a coworker dropping by to chat, or urgent tasks demanding attention can disrupt your workflow and shift your focus away from what you were originally working on.

5. **Internal distractions:** Sometimes distractions come from within. Intrusive thoughts: worries or personal concerns can occupy our minds and make it challenging to concentrate on the task at hand. Keep a small notebook handy so that you can take your worries from your head to the paper. Having it written down frees up space in your mind.

When you feel stuck, and we all do (Lord knows how many

times I was completely stuck writing this book), step away and take a walk around the block, listen to music. Come back with a fresh perspective.

Next, take action. As humans we get caught up in our heads and thoughts and never get past that. The antidote is to do *something*. And that something is to act.

1. **Put it on paper:** Take pen and paper and write down what you need to accomplish today. Number them in sequence of importance.

2. **Find a comfortable, distraction free workspace:** I have been known to go to the library and hole up in one of their (free) study rooms. I schedule breaks to avoid burnout. My phone will get me off course in a New York minute, so I put it on *Do Not Disturb*. I avoid surfing the Web, Amazon, social media, as these can be a black hole. I stay focused on the task at hand and really dive into it.

3. **Check items off your list:** Nothing feels as good as checking items off your list. Doing this shows that you are making strides and getting things done. Ultimately, this will lead you closer and closer to your goals.

4. **Pat myself on the back:** Once I have accomplished my tasks, I pat myself on the back and carry on with my day. Acknowledging your progress goes a long way.

Lather, rinse, repeat!

EXERCISE

Some of my distractions are:

1. Shopping.

2. Eating (Admit it, you've gone to that refrigerator more than once to find the same food there each time: own up, there's no shame in the game).

3. Talking and texting on the phone.

What are your distractions:

1.

2.

3.

I am ready.
I am available.
Show me how.

Notes

Notes

CHAPTER 11
Procrastination

"Procrastination is like a credit card:
it's a lot of fun until you get the bill."
—Christopher Parker

THIS IS A BIG ONE, PEOPLE! PUTTING OFF UNTIL TOMOR-
row what can be done today. Didn't you hate when you were a
kid and your parents said, "Never put off until tomorrow what
you can do today." I know I did.

Procrastination often involves engaging in activities that
provide immediate gratification or are more enjoyable than the
task we should be working on. I'm guilty of this and I hear
many people say they are as well. It's a tough one but keep your
eye on the prize and keep going.

The secret of getting ahead is getting started. Procrastinating, or delaying what needs to be done, just puts you behind
the eight ball. But I get it. Sometimes things seem so overwhelming that you can't decide where to start. Write down
three things you need to do. Pick one task and just start.

I wish I could give you a cure for procrastination but the
best I can do is to share some actionable steps that I use to help
me overcome procrastinating:

1. **Worst things first:** I had a real estate coach that
   always said this, and it makes perfect sense. If you
   tackle the least favorite task first, you are good to
   go. You don't have to dread it all day. Knock it out
   early and get on with other activities.

2. **Make a list:** At night, I make a list of what I want/
   need to accomplish tomorrow. Then I prioritize my
   list and schedule an allotted amount of time for

each task. I take out my list in the morning and reassess it, making sure the priorities I set yesterday still make sense today.

3. **Put your nose to the grindstone:** Life is like a grindstone; whether it grinds you down or polishes you up depends on you. Get to that list now!

Time is a non-renewable resource. Don't waste it!

EXERCISE

I will eliminate procrastination today by:

1) Knocking out the task I dread the most first.

2) Staying in action.

3) Turning off my cellular devices.

Now your turn:

1.

2.

3.

I am ready.
I am available.
Show me how.

Notes

CHAPTER 12
Buh-Bye Limiting Beliefs

*"You begin to fly when you let go of self-limiting beliefs
and allow your mind and aspirations
to rise to greater heights."*
—Brian Tracy

WHAT ARE LIMITING BELIEFS? A LIMITING BELIEF IS A state of mind or belief about yourself that restricts you in some way. These beliefs are often false accusations you make about yourself that can cause a number of negative results. Do not, I repeat, do not let your self-limiting beliefs get in the way of your greatness.

Here are a few examples of common self-limiting beliefs:

1. **I'm not smart/talented enough:** Believing that you lack intelligence or talent can prevent you from pursuing new opportunities or challenging yourself intellectually.

2. **I don't deserve success:** Feeling unworthy of success can lead to self-sabotaging behaviors and prevent you from fully embracing and achieving your goals.

3. **I'm too old:** Hey, Colonel Sanders of Kentucky Fried Chicken began franchising his chicken business at the age of 65 and sold it at the age of 73. It's never too late.

4. **I'm too young:** No such thing. Mark Zuckerberg started Facebook when he was a mere 19 years old.

5. **I'm not good with money:** This belief can create financial insecurity and prevent you from developing healthy financial habits or seeking opportunities

for wealth creation. There is so much information out there to educate yourself. Suze Orman, financial advisor, author, and podcast host, has a wealth (pun intended) of information out there to educate yourself in all financial matters. Or better yet, hire a financial planner. They are a great resource. Ask your bank if they have one on staff.

Can you relate to any or all of these? Most of us can and do. But overcoming limiting beliefs is crucial for personal development and achieving success.

Here are some strategies to challenge and overcome self-limiting beliefs:

1. **Self-awareness:** Recognize and identify the limiting beliefs that are holding you back. Understand how they impact your thoughts, emotions, and actions.

2. **Question that belief:** Challenge the validity of your limiting beliefs by questioning the evidence supporting them. Seek alternative perspectives and evidence that contradicts these beliefs. Check out Byron Katie, speaker and author, who teaches a method of self-inquiry known as "The Work."

3. **Reframe and reprogram:** Replace negative, limiting beliefs with positive and empowering ones. Practice affirmations, positive self-talk, and visualization to rewire your mindset.

4. **Take action:** Actively pursue activities and goals that challenge your limiting beliefs. Start with small steps and gradually push yourself outside of

your comfort zone.

5. **Seek support:** Surround yourself with positive and supportive people who can encourage and inspire you. Consider working with a therapist, coach, or mentor who can provide guidance and help you navigate through limiting beliefs.

Remember, overcoming limiting beliefs is a process that requires time, effort, and persistence. With dedication and a growth mindset, you can break free from these self-imposed limitations and unlock your full potential.

So, let go of your self-limiting beliefs and go for it! Really go for it! What do you have to lose? The world is your oyster. You can have anything you want in life or go anywhere you want because you have the opportunity or ability to do so!

'Nuff said!

EXERCISE

Some of my limiting beliefs are:

1. I don't have enough time. You can make more time in your day by making a daily routine and following it.

2. I'm not smart enough. Says who? If they can do it, so can I.

3. I can't do this. Of course you can. Break it down into bite-size pieces and just start.

List three limiting beliefs you have and how you plan to overcome them:

1.

2.

3.

I am ready.
I am available.
Show me how.

Notes

Notes

CHAPTER 13
Compare and Despair

*"I always say my biggest competitor is myself because,
whenever I step out there on the mat,
I'm competing against myself to prove that I can do this
and that I am very well trained, prepared for it."*
—Simone Biles

IT NEVER CEASES TO AMAZE ME HOW MANY PEOPLE compare themselves to others (and to be transparent, I have fallen into this category on more than one occasion). And truth be told, there is always going to be someone prettier, thinner, richer, smarter, etc. But life is not meant to be a competition. We were all put on earth with our own special gifts to share with the world.

To compare and despair describes the tendency to compare oneself unfavorably to others, leading to feelings of dissatisfaction, envy, and low self-esteem.

Let's break it down:

1. **Compare:** Comparing is the act of assessing similarities and differences between two or more things or people. It's a natural human tendency to compare ourselves to others in various aspects such as appearance, success, intelligence, wealth, or relationships. But it gets you nowhere. Focus on *you* and being the best *you* that you can be.

2. **Despair:** Despair refers to a state of hopelessness, discouragement, or deep sadness. When you engage in constant comparison and find yourself falling short or feeling inferior, it can lead to feelings of despair and a negative self-perception. Remember we all have our special abilities and talents.

When combined, compare and despair represents the negative emotional state that arises from consistently comparing oneself to others and feeling inadequate as a result.

It's important to note that comparison itself is not inherently negative. It can be useful for self-reflection, motivation, and personal growth when approached in a healthy and constructive manner. However, when comparisons become obsessive or lead to self-criticism and despair, they can have detrimental effects on one's well-being. In short, don't do it!

You are not meant to live as others. You are meant to live as yourself. We're all cut from a different cloth. Personally, I was never cut out for corporate America. Sitting at a desk from nine to five just never did it for me. Do I sometimes wonder if that would have been an easier path? Of course I do. But I chose not to go down that road. I march to the beat of a different drummer.

To overcome this compare and despair mindset, it is helpful to focus on self-acceptance, gratitude, and personal progress rather than constantly measuring oneself against others. Embracing individuality, setting realistic goals, and developing self-compassion are effective strategies for cultivating a positive self-image and reducing the negative impact of comparisons.

When you compare your insides to someone else's outsides, you are going to come up short nine times out of ten. Instead celebrate yourself, celebrate others. Revel in their success. Do not be envious. Remember if they can do it, so can you. It's a big world. There's room for everyone.

My mom always told me that if you had a room full of people, and everyone put their problems in a pile in the middle of the room, we'd grab our own problems back. Everyone is fighting some kind of battle. Focus on you! Be the best *you* that you can possibly be. Resist the urge to compare. It gets you nowhere fast.

Now get out there and shine your bright, beautiful, and unique light!

EXERCISE

Here are three truths I remember when I compare and despair:

1. Social media is glamorized.

2. You have no idea what they went through to get where they are.

3. If they can do it, so can I.

Now your turn:

1.

2.

3.

I am ready.
I am available.
Show me how.

Notes

Notes

CHAPTER 14
Unplug

"All work and no play make Jack a dull boy."
—Proverb
—Famous line by Jack Nicholson in the movie *The Shining*

WE ALL KNOW THAT WHEN WE HAVE A PROBLEM WITH our electronics, phone, TV, computer, the go-to solution is to unplug it, let it sit a few seconds, and then plug it back in. Sometimes that is the fix that is needed. We, as humans, also need to unplug.

Breaks are important. Not taking enough breaks leads to burnout, and higher stress levels. Taking periodic work breaks can boost well-being and performance but far too few of us take them. According to Aflac, more than half of employees (59%) report feeling burnout. Taking breaks increases productivity, improves mental health and well-being, can prevent decision fatigue, and increases creativity, to name just a few of the benefits.

In this go, go, go culture that we live in, the concept of taking a break is oftentimes looked down upon, and being a workaholic is praised. This seems so backward. How do you feel after you get away from your desk, even just to step outside and take some deep breaths? For me, a break from work is as important as the work itself. I can get so caught up in my writing that I forget to take a break. My husband reminds me almost every day. I get into a rhythm and don't want to stop. But getting my mind off work and stepping away actually increases my productivity, fuels my creativity, and just makes me happier all around. Nine times out of ten my creativity and productivity improve immensely when I step away.

How often should you take a break? And how long should your breaks last? There are many schools of thought concerning the optimal timing of breaks. The trick is finding the right break schedule for your work style. Experiment with taking a break every 30 to 90 minutes until you learn what is best for you. Then schedule breaks on your calendar or in your planner and stick to them.

To make your break productive, you need to do something completely different from your work, and something that you enjoy. Here are just a few ways to take a break and recharge your mind:

1. **Physical activity:** Go for a walk, do some stretching exercises, or engage in any form of physical activity that you enjoy. It can help improve blood circulation and boost your energy to boot.

2. **Spend time in nature:** Go to a park, a garden, or any outdoor setting that allows you to relax and enjoy the beauty of nature. Fresh air and natural surroundings can have a calming effect on the mind.

3. **Disconnect from technology:** Spend some time away from screens. Put away your phone, computer, or any other electronic devices. Engage in activities that don't require technology, such as reading a book or eating a healthy snack. My go-to is an apple with peanut butter.

4. **Socialize:** Spend time with family or friends. Meet up for a coffee, have a great conversation, or engage in an activity together. Socializing can provide a mental break and help you feel rejuvenated. Try it.

5. **Pursue a hobby:** Make time to do what you love and are passionate about. It could be painting, playing an instrument, cooking, gardening, or any other hobby that brings you joy. I love to Google different plant-based recipes and make my own healthy dinner.

6. **Laugh:** Watch a funny video, listen to your favorite comedian on YouTube. My favorite comedian right now is Sebastian Maniscalco. Check him out. Researchers from Finland and the United Kingdom found that social laughter triggers the release of endorphins—often referred to as "feel-good hormones"—in brain regions responsible for arousal and emotion (Medical News Today).

7. **Listen to your favorite music:** Listening to music can reduce anxiety, blood pressure, and pain, as well as improve sleep quality, mood, mental alertness, and memory. So, plug in those ear pods/AirPods and listen to your favorite music. I'm a country music fan myself. Can't get enough of it.

8. **Eat a healthy snack:** I don't mean hitting the vending machines at work. Consider these simple and nourishing options. Greek yogurt with berries, apple slices with nut butter, veggie sticks with hummus. Sometimes a little snack is the pick-me-up you may be needing.

Remember, breaks are essential for maintaining balance and preventing burnout. Listen to your body, take breaks when you need them, and return to your task with renewed energy and focus.

EXERCISE

What are three activities you can do today on your breaks? I'll start:

1. Take a walk around the block.

2. Watch something funny and laugh out loud.

3. Refuel with a healthy snack.

Now your turn:

1.

2.

3.

I am ready.
I am available.
Show me how.

Notes

Notes

CHAPTER 15
Mental Gym, Work It Out

"The mind is just like a muscle — the more you exercise it, the stronger it gets and the more it can expand."
—Idowu Koyenikan

I THINK WE ALL KNOW THE BENEFITS OF KEEPING OUR physical bodies in shape, but what about our minds? Your mind is like a muscle. You've got to visit the mental gym daily to keep it sharp. After all, you wouldn't go to the gym every day, stop going, and expect the results to last. Same is true for the mental gym.

You may be asking "What the heck is a mental gym?" Meditation, gratitude, yoga, breathing exercises, daily affirmations, reading, journaling, listening to or watching inspirational podcasts or videos, are just some of the tools in the mental gym. By practicing any, or all these modalities on a daily basis, you will keep your mind in tip-top shape. And a strong mindset leads to a happy and more positive mood. And to top it off, researchers have discovered neuroplasticity, which is the brain's ability to change itself constantly by creating new neural pathways and losing those which are no longer used.

Let's take a deep dive into a few of these and find out how they can benefit you:

1. **Gratitude** for all the blessings in your life is essential. Focusing on what's good in our lives and being thankful for the things we have.

   "I cried because I had no shoes
   until I saw a man who had no feet."

   Be grateful for what you have because someone always has it worse. Count your blessings. Pause to notice and appreciate the things that we often take for granted, like having a place to live, good food, clean water, friends, family, even computer access.

After all, where would we be without our computers? Get into a practice of making a list every day of what you are grateful for. It doesn't have to be a long list. Even just two to three things. Don't overwhelm yourself. Once you start you may find that many more come to mind.

2. **Meditation** is a simple practice available to us all. It can reduce stress, increase calmness and clarity, and promote happiness. And the best thing is you don't need any fancy equipment to get started. Simply find a place to sit that feels calm and quiet to you. Set a time limit. I recommend 10 to 20 minutes but do what feels comfortable to you. Close your eyes, feel your breath. Inevitably your mind will wander. Don't judge yourself. Simply return your attention to your breath.

   Having a hard time getting started? Try using a meditation app. Just Google meditation apps and you will find a plethora of them. Two of my favorites are CALM and HEADSPACE. Apps are especially great for beginners. Give it a shot.

3. **Yoga** has become very mainstream in recent years. Personally, I love yoga and have practiced for many years. Yoga is a complete workout for both mind and body. It is not only a powerful way to relax

but increases fat loss, develops muscle tone, and builds flexibility, leading to a more toned body and a peaceful mind. Yoga studios are popping up everywhere, but if you cannot find one near you, you can always stay at home and do a video. There are tens of thousands of yoga videos. So, give it a try. As little as 10 to 20 minutes a day and you will feel the difference.

4. **Breathwork** is trending right now but it's not new. People have been practicing breathwork for thousands of years. The basic idea is to inhale deeply to nourish your mind and body, and exhale to release toxins and stress. When you feel stressed, your breath tends to become fast and shallow, limiting the amount of oxygen entering your bloodstream. When you slow down and purposely breathe deep and slow, you send a message to your brain that everything is OK. So, stop what you are doing and take ten slow, deep breaths in and out. Feel the difference?

5. **Affirmations** are positive statements that can help brighten your outlook on the world when you say them to yourself regularly or write them down. If you're looking to form better mental health habits, this is a great (and free) place to start. I keep my affirmations in clear sight by writing them on an index card, posting them on my bulletin board, taping them to a mirror, and to the dashboard in my car.

EXERCISE

Here are a few of my favorite affirmations:

1. I am in the right place at the right time, doing the right thing.

2. I am powerful, and my life is about to become even more incredible.

3. I must do the things I think I cannot do.

List three affirmations that speak to your soul:

1.

2.

3.

I am ready.
I am available.
Show me how.

Notes

Notes

CHAPTER 16
Who Do You Think You Are?
Seriously, Who Are You?

"I am strong beyond belief. I am powerful beyond measure."
—Marianne Williamson

WE ALL HAVE STORIES WE BELIEVE ABOUT OURSELVES. What story are you telling yourself? Is it serving you? Is it enhancing your life, or bringing you down? Do you want to change that story? Do you believe you can? Some of us have been carrying the same story around since childhood. Stop that. If your story is not serving you, change it!

Hopefully by reading this book, you have been able to take a deep dive and really think about your life. Are you happy? Are you fulfilled? If you are, great! If not, let's figure out why and take the steps to change your story to an empowering, life-affirming story.

Here are a few things you can do to change your story in a positive direction:

1. **Surround yourself with positive people**: You are the sum of who you surround yourself with. Choose to spend time with positive and supportive individuals. A positive social environment can have a significant impact on your mindset.

2. **Challenge yourself**: Step out of your comfort zone and take on new challenges. Overcoming obstacles can boost confidence and resilience.

3. **Do something different**: As the saying goes, "Keep doing what you're doing, keep getting what you're getting." Try something different. Always wanted

to ride a horse? Do it. Want to snowboard? Try it.

4. **Keep a journal:** There is something very cathartic about keeping a journal. Journaling can stimulate creativity. Free flow writing or creative exercises in a journal can inspire new ideas and perspectives.

You can rewrite your story anytime!

EXERCISE

My "I am" statements:

1) I am Confident!

2) I am Fearless!

3) I am Powerful!

Who are *you*:

1.

2.

3.

I am ready.
I am available.
Show me how.

Notes

CHAPTER 17
Lights, Camera, Action!

"An object in rest tends to stay in rest.
An object in motion tends to stay in motion."
—Sir Isaac Newton

TIME TO TAKE ACTION. ACTION BREEDS CONFIDENCE and courage. Inaction breeds doubt and fear.

We can heed the words of Teddy Roosevelt's "*The Man in the Arena.*"

"It is not the critic who counts; not the man who points out how the strong man stumbles, or where the doer of deeds could have done them better. The credit belongs to the man who is actually in the arena, whose face is marred by dust and sweat and blood; who strives valiantly; who errs, who comes short again and again, because there is no effort without error and shortcoming; but who does actually strive to do the deeds; who knows great enthusiasms, the great devotions; who spends himself in a worthy cause; who at the best knows in the end the triumph of high achievement, and who at the worst, if he fails, at least fails while daring greatly, so that his place shall never be with those cold and timid souls who neither know victory nor defeat."

I don't care how small or insignificant the action may be. As Nike says, "*Just Do It!*" One action will lead to the next, and, before you know it, you are on your way. Taking action is a crucial step toward achieving your goals and making positive changes in your life. Whether you want to pursue a new career, improve your health and fitness, learn a new skill, or start your own business, here are some tips to get you into action:

1. **Take the first step:** The journey of a thousand miles begins with a single step.

   The hardest part of any journey is the first step. Once you take that initial step, you're sure to gain momentum. Keep moving forward.

2. **Set clear goals:** Define what you want to achieve. Make sure your goals are S.M.A.R.T: Specific, Measurable, Achievable, Relevant, and Time-bound.

3. **Feeling listless, make a list:** One of the most significant benefits of making a list is that it will help you stay organized. It also helps those tasks appear more manageable. You'll be able to stay more focused because you've got an outline of what you've got to do and things you've already completed.

4. **Keep it simple:** Heed the acronym K.I.S.S. Keep It Simple Stupid. No reason to make things harder than they have to be. Aim for simplicity.

By now you should have identified some clear, actionable steps you can take right now. Get into action and start making your dreams a reality.

And remember, keep it simple.

I leave you with lights-camera-action! Now go out there and get 'er done!

EXERCISE

I will stay in action by:

1. Writing, writing, writing.

2. Exercising.

3. Brainstorming my next book.

What are three things you can do right now to get into action:

1.

2.

3.

I am ready.
I am available.
Show me how.

Notes

CHAPTER 18
Who Is This Betsy Mendel?

"I've lived a life that's full
I traveled each and every highway.
And more, much more than this
I did it my way."
—Frank Sinatra

BY NOW YOU MAY BE WONDERING "WHO THE HECK IS this Betsy Mendel?" As you can see, I don't have any letters before or after my name, nor am I a famous writer (yet). But I will tell you, that is my goal.

My credentials are life, 64 rotations around the sun have given me my share of experience and wisdom.

I've always marched to the beat of a different drummer. To quote Henry David Thoreau's 1854 work, *Walden*:

"If a man does not keep pace with his companions, perhaps it is because he hears a different drummer. Let him step to the music he hears, however measured or far away."

I would like to share the music I have heard during my time on this planet. I have had many careers and experiences which have shaped me into who I am today.

First off, a little about me. I was born and raised in Atlanta, Georgia and now reside in sunny Santa Monica, California with my husband, Rick, and my cat, Patches, who really runs the show. It's her world and we just live in it. Living just ten blocks from the beach you can catch me taking "the plunge" in the cold Pacific Ocean! Talk about invigorating. With the Santa Monica Mountains just minutes from my door, I hike every Saturday. Along with all that, I am at the gym five days a week to get my daily dose of endorphins: my saving grace. I consider myself a foodie, but my friends would argue there is no such thing as a vegan(ish) foodie. I love dining out at all the great and healthy restaurants Los Angeles has to offer and enjoying a nice glass of vino (or two).

Now on to all the varied and colorful careers:

My very first job was as a waitress, working my way through college (shocker, I know).

Next, I did my stint as a model. My favorite gig was modeling self-tanning lotion when it first came out in the '80s. Lancôme was the first on board. I was hired by Saks Fifth Avenue in Atlanta to put the self-tanning lotion on only one side of my body. I picked out a bikini and stood in the makeshift beach scene they had created in the store. I'm very fair so the contrast was quite amazing. Needless to say, many bottles of self-tanner were sold. Fast forward to today where all we have to do is step in a booth, and we can come out tan in just minutes. Now that's what I call innovation.

After that, I went to work for an international marketing company running promotions for 4- and 5-star hotels. I traveled to many cities with this job. One of my favorite cities was Breckenridge, Colorado. I had never been to a ski resort before. I immediately fell in love with skiing and everything about the lifestyle. I fantasized about moving there, and lo and behold, one day I was getting fitted for my ski boots and I happened to mention that I would love to live out here. Well, I manifested that quickly. The guy helping me out said he happens to have an extra bedroom that he needs to rent (remember this is the '80s). So back to Atlanta I went, packed my bags, and moved to Breckenridge (ahhh, youth) where I enjoyed life as a ski bum for two winters. By the way, I recommend this to anyone in their twenties. Experience another part of the country while you are still young.

From there it was back to Atlanta where I had no clue what

my next move was going to be. Hold tight. This one's a real doozie. My mom knew of a woman in Savannah whose daughter started catering to car dealerships with sandwiches and desserts. So, I put on my best apron, filled my basket with sandwiches, chips, and desserts, and off I went. Right away I was a hit. So, I decided to start my own catering business, "Heavens to Betsy, Out of This World Catering." From chicken salad sandwiches to Devil's food cake and Angel food cake, I was on my way. Sidenote: I was rumored to have the best chicken salad in the city, which is quite funny as I don't eat chicken, so I never tasted it myself. I started calling on stock brokerage firms which became a perfect match as they have lunch meetings all the time. From there, it just grew, but I was not loving it. It was too much work for too little return. So, I retired my apron and went back to the drawing board.

I was feeling a bit restless, and I always dreamed of living in California. The same company that led me to Breckenridge resurfaced and put me back on the road. From Dallas to Utah to Los Angeles, I was loving life. I got to scratch my travel itch and get paid to do it. Leave it to me, when I arrived in Los Angeles, I knew I had to spend some time here. The company I was working for started having financial problems and I found myself unemployed. But not to worry. My brother, who is a dentist on the East Coast, knew of a dental company looking for inside salespeople in Los Angeles. So, you guessed it, I went to work selling dental products. Dr. Bill Dorfman of *Extreme Makeover* fame owned the company. This is the early 2000's and teeth whitening was all the rage.

Although I was very successful in my job, I wanted my own company. I have always had an entrepreneurial spirit and was never cut out for the nine to five grind. Soooo . . . my friend

Rachel and I started a T-shirt company, "Awareables, You Are What You Wear." We combined our creative juices along with Rachel's experience as a fashion designer for Warner Brothers. We came up with witty sayings such as "There's No Place Like Om," "Gratitude Rocks," "Inhale, Exhale, Repeat," "Namaste Namasgo," and "Shift Happens" to name a few. We had a fabulous product and had some success, but in the end, we did not know how to scale it, so we hung up our T-shirt line.

Now this is my sweet spot: personal trainer. I have always worked out and followed a healthy diet. My discipline and devotion to a healthy lifestyle is something that has always come super easily to me. From running cross-country in high school to the aerobics boom in the '80s to power yoga to spinning, I have done it all. And at 64 years old, I think my hard work has paid off in spades. I look and feel (and act) decades younger. I still have my training business today and still love helping people reach their full fitness potential.

As much as I absolutely love guiding people on their path to a healthy lifestyle, I was still struggling to make ends meet, which leads me to my next career . . .

When all else fails, get your real estate license. I mean really, where else can you make boatloads of money working on your own schedule and having fun to boot . . . NOT! Real estate agents look like they are raking in the moolah, and many are, but looks can be deceiving. The National Association of Realtors (NAR) found that 75% of realtors fail within the first year of being in the industry and 87% after five years. Unfortunately, I became part of that statistic. After four years, I realized real estate was not a good fit for me. But no regrets as I gained so much knowledge and made some great friends along the way. There is always a bright side to every story.

And finally, today I am a health and wellness coach for an international weight-loss, weight-management, and nutrition company as well as a private personal trainer. I love combining nutrition and physical activity with counseling to help clients change their lifestyle and eating habits. I enjoy this job immensely and it comes very naturally to me. I love coaching people to follow a healthy lifestyle. My job is to help people live their best life ever. And really, when it comes down to it, what could be better than that!

But through all the years and careers, the one thing that has always been a constant in my life is my desire to write. Intuitively, I knew I should be writing. Hence, this book.

So, as you can see, I've had a varied and colorful life which has shaped me into who I am today. I chose the road less traveled. You do what suits *you*.

If you have read this far, I want to thank you from the bottom of my heart for reading my book. I wish you all the success the world has to offer, however that may look for you.

And hey, to quote Zig Ziglar, "I'll see you at the top."

Notes

CHAPTER 19
Betsy's Best Bets

"If you never did, you should.
These things are fun, and fun is good."
—Dr. Seuss

AT 64, I FEEL HALF MY AGE. IN NO PARTICULAR ORDER, I want to share with you secrets that have helped me over the years on this journey called life. I hope you can use some or all of these. Enjoy!

MAKE YOUR BED:

Admiral William H. McRaven, Retired Navy SEAL, speaker and author writes in his #1 New York Times Bestseller, *Make Your Bed – Little Things That Can Change Your Life . . . And Maybe the World*. McRaven tells us "If you make your bed every morning, you will have accomplished the first task of the day. It will give you a sense of pride, and it will encourage you to do another task and another and another. By the end of the day, that one task completed will have turned into many tasks completed. Making your bed will also reinforce the fact that little things in life matter. If you can't do the little things right, you will never be able to do the big things right."

MOVE YOUR BODY EVERY DAY
LAUGH
EAT PLANT-BASED AS MUCH AS POSSIBLE
BE KIND TO YOURSELF
BE KIND TO OTHERS
COMPLIMENT ONE PERSON A DAY
DON'T SWEAT THE SMALL STUFF
DON'T SMOKE
EVERYTHING IN MODERATION

USE SUNSCREEN

CHOOSE YOUR BATTLES WISELY

WEAR POLARIZED SUNGLASSES

PLAY WITH YOUR PET

SMILE!

LISTEN TO YOUR BODY

RETURN TEXTS PROMPTLY

MAKE EVERYDAY COUNT

NEVER SAY NEVER

NEVER, EVER COMPARE

HANG IN THERE:

Feelings are much like waves, we can't stop them from coming, but we can choose which ones to surf.

WHEN IN DOUBT . . . GOOGLE

GET A YEARLY CHECKUP FROM YOUR DOCTOR

PEN AND PAPER BY BED

TIME BLOCK

DRINK PLENTY OF WATER DAILY:

64oz. works for me. The general rule is to drink one ounce of water for every two pounds of body weight.

CHOOSE YOUR FRIENDS WISELY:

You are the sum of who you surround yourself with.

TECHNOLOGY: Master one new thing a week.

SOAK IN A WARM EPSOM SALT BATH

NEVER GHOST ANYONE

READ TEN PAGES OF SOMETHING EVERY DAY

FLOSS

MEDITATE: Even five minutes has its benefits.

FALL IN LOVE WITH YOURSELF

BUY YOURSELF SOME FLOWERS

AND FINALLY: *CALL YOUR MOTHER!*

EXERCISE:

I've shared my favorite tips with you. Now it's time for you to write yours:

1.

2.

3.

I am ready.
I am available.
Show me how.

Notes

CHAPTER 20
Your Dream Life

"The world's mine oyster."
—Shakespeare

YOUR TURN. TIME TO PUT PEN TO PAPER. USE THE BLANK pages that follow to write your dream life. Write it as if you are already living it. Have fun!

EXERCISE:

Three things that bring me joy:

1. Jumping in the ocean.

2. Eating at my favorite restaurant.

3. Connecting with friends.

Your three things:

1.

2.

3.

Now pat yourself on the back and go out and do something that brings you joy!

I am ready.
I am available.
Show me how.

My Life

EPILOGUE

*"Everything will be OK in the end.
If it's not OK, it's not the end."*
—Unknown

OKAY PEOPLE. TIME TO HAVE A HEART TO HEART. YOU'VE read my book. Hopefully you've completed the exercises at the end of each chapter. Now what? Are you ready to say buh-bye to mediocrity and hello to awesomeness? Starting right now!

Truth be told, I wrote *Buh-Bye Mediocrity, Hello Awesomeness!* as much for myself as for you. My heartfelt wish is for you to really, really, really get it, apply what you have learned, and soar to new heights.

Remember how I told you that this book is written in bite-size pieces? Take what resonates with you, savor it, digest it. Come back for seconds and thirds and on and on.

I believe in you. You've so got this!!!

ACKNOWLEDGEMENTS

To my amazingly awesome husband, Rick. I could never have written this book without your unwavering support and encouragement. Thank you for inspiring me to embrace my awesomeness and for sharing your invaluable wisdom with me.

It takes a village. A heartfelt thanks to all my amazing friends who have kept me on this journey and stayed with me to the finish line. A special thanks to Jon Gordon for the amazing endorsement. Thank you Kathryn Gordon for the beautiful Foreword. Cindy Stern, you actually sat there and listened to me read every single page of the book. Your insights have made such a difference. Thank you! Lauren Foster, you never complained when I sent you attachment after attachment with all the changes. You helped me find my voice. Joyce Stein, you are my biggest cheerleader! Thanks for believing in me and assuring me I am on the right path. Rachel Layne, what can I say. I'll never forget when you read the manuscript and the first thing out of your mouth was "I have got to get this book."

Additionally, shout out to Sandra Steinbook and Nancy King who so generously opened their homes to me when I traveled to Atlanta, giving me the space I needed to really write.

Without you guys I don't think this book would have come to fruition. Much love!

Thank you to my editor, Roseanna M. White. Your guidance and expertise have been invaluable!

Thank you to my IT guru, Zakir Alibhai. Without you I would have used a stone tablet and a chisel. You were a godsend. Thank you!

And lastly, my cat Patches, who just makes me smile every day.

Thank you all for being a part of this awesome journey.

With gratitude,

Betsy

Amazingly Awesome Betsy!

ABOUT BETSY

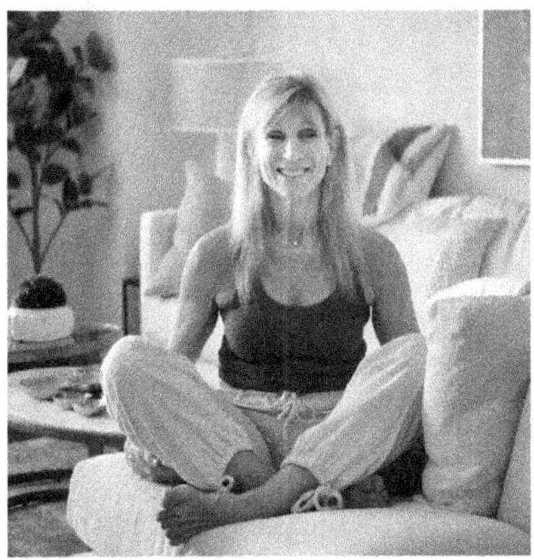

Originally from Atlanta, GA, Betsy moved to California in search of a lifestyle change. Her dedication to health and fitness brought her to Santa Monica, where she quickly immersed herself in activities like biking, hiking, hot yoga, spin classes, and HIIT. She channeled her passion for a healthy lifestyle into helping others look and feel their best.

Her sweet spot is the beach, where she's known to plunge into the cold Pacific Ocean anytime, including the polar plunge on New Year's Day. Betsy jokes that she might have been a fish in a past life! After a day at the beach, you'll find her sipping an Aperol Spritz at one of her favorite patio bars.

Betsy's passion lies in empowering others to break free from mediocrity and embrace an amazingly awesome life!

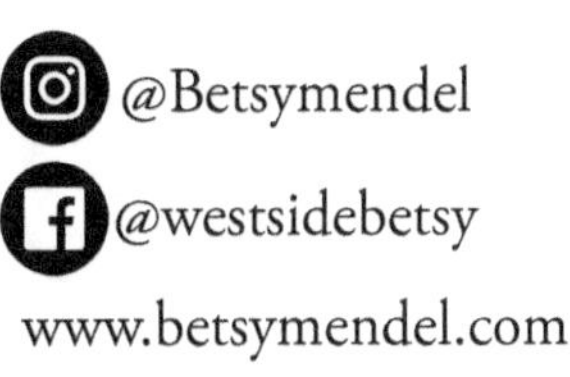

www.betsymendel.com

www.ingramcontent.com/pod-product-compliance
Lightning Source LLC
Chambersburg PA
CBHW071433130726
47997CB00006B/2070